THE LOW CHOLESTEROL COOKBOOK AND ACTION PLAN

Heart-Healthy Eating Made Easy with Delicious and Nutritious Recipes

Kimberly Williams J.

Related books:

Low Cholesterol Dessert Cookbook

https://www.amazon.com/dp/B0CKYH9VGB

TABLE OF CONTENTS

Introduction

A vital component of our general well-being, heart health is essential to living a long and happy life. The human heart is the engine that maintains our bodies functioning properly because of its continuous rhythm. Realizing the value of heart health is about preserving the quality of the years we have left, not just about how long we live. This introduction emphasizes why heart health is an area that requires our attention and care, setting the basis for a deeper exploration of its essential components.

Overview of Heart Health's Significance

As a muscle that never stops, our heart pumps blood throughout our bodies, supplying each and every cell with vital nutrients and oxygen. The heart and blood vessels make up the cardiovascular system, which is a sophisticated network essential to the body's overall operation. An effective circulatory system, which supports optimal organ function and general vigor, is synonymous with a healthy heart.

Heart health refers to the state of this important organ as well as the network that supports it. Cardiovascular diseases continue to be a major cause of death globally, but they are less likely to occur in people with healthy hearts. excessive blood pressure, excessive cholesterol, and a sedentary lifestyle are just a few of the variables that can negatively impact heart health and lead to conditions including coronary artery disease, heart attacks, and strokes.

In addition to preventing disease, maintaining heart health also involves creating an atmosphere that supports the heart's growth. Better mental clarity, more vitality, and a stronger sense of wellbeing are all influenced by a healthy heart. It makes it possible for people to live active lives, follow their passions, and take delight in the small things in life that bring great fulfilment.

It is clear that taking care of our hearts is an investment in our future as we learn more about the significance of heart health. It's a dedication to living a longer, healthier life and being able to fully appreciate each moment.

The Difficulty of Developing a Heart-Healthy Nutrition

Although there is no denying the importance of heart health, many people find it difficult to lead heart-healthy lives. Making deliberate decisions that put our hearts' well-being first takes work and commitment in a world full with mouthwatering food and hectic lifestyles.

A major obstacle that people have is navigating a dietary landscape that may not always follow heart-healthy guidelines. The "bad" cholesterol, or LDL cholesterol, is frequently raised in modern diets because they are heavy in cholesterol, trans fats, and saturated fats. This may result in an accumulation of plaque in the arteries, raising the possibility of developing heart disease.

People find it more difficult to strike a balance between their dietary needs and the demands of a busy lifestyle. In a society where efficiency and speed are highly valued, processed and convenience foods—which are frequently loaded with unhealthy fats and sodium—can seem like sensible options. It takes dedication and persistence to break free from these behaviors since it is a conscious decision to put health before convenience.

Furthermore, a heart-healthy diet calls for embracing a wide variety of nutrient-rich foods in addition to avoiding particular ones. This entails including entire grains, lean meats, fruits, and veggies in every meal. The change can be faced with resistance and doubt from people who are not used to such eating practices.

Changing our eating habits is only one aspect of the issue of implementing a heart-healthy diet; another is rethinking our connection with food. It necessitates conscious eating, knowledge of dietary options, and comprehension of how those options affect our heart health. Planning, education, and a willingness to try new foods and cooking methods are all necessary for this transition.

Comprehending the Effects of Cholesterol

Gaining knowledge about cholesterol is essential to enhancing heart health. Blood contains a type of fat called cholesterol. While our bodies require some cholesterol to function properly, excessive amounts of cholesterol can be hazardous. LDL (bad) and HDL (good) cholesterol are the two primary types. LDL cholesterol raises the risk of heart disease by clogging the arteries with accumulation. Conversely, HDL cholesterol lowers the risk by assisting in the removal of LDL cholesterol from the bloodstream. You can make educated decisions about your diet and way of life by becoming knowledgeable about these kinds and how they impact your health.

Professional Advice for Grocery Shopping and Meal Planning

There are some important things to remember when grocery shopping for foods that are heart-healthy. Prioritize fresh produce, whole grains, lean meats like chicken and fish, and fresh fruits and vegetables first. As processed foods are heavy in trans and saturated fats and can increase LDL cholesterol, try to stay away from them. You may make better decisions and find hidden fats by reading food labels. Making a grocery list based on these recommendations can help you shop more efficiently and guarantee that you have everything you need for heart-healthy meals prepared at home.

Including Frequent Exercise to Promote Heart Health

Enhancing heart health requires regular exercise. Regular physical activity can help lower LDL cholesterol levels and raise HDL cholesterol levels. It doesn't have to be strenuous - even moderate exercise like brisk walking, swimming, or cycling can make a major effect. Aim for at least 30 minutes of activity most days of the week. Incorporating exercise into your regimen not only benefits your heart but also boosts your entire well-being. Start with baby steps and progressively improve your activity level for a healthier heart.

The 4-Week Action Plan

First Week: Establishing the Base

Starting the transition to a heart-healthy lifestyle needs to be done thoughtfully and with knowledge. During the first week, you will be fully engaged in introspection, examining your present routines and creating a detailed plan for the upcoming weeks. Here is a thorough analysis of Week 1's key components:

Evaluating Present Food Practices

Start by examining your present eating patterns in detail. This entails a careful analysis of the foods, snacks, and drinks you consume each day. This is not a judging exercise; rather, it is meant to foster knowledge and understanding.

Make use of the available tools and resources to record and monitor your eating habits with precision. This examination will provide important information about your eating patterns. Do you eat too much added sugar or saturated fat? Do you eat enough fruits, veggies, and whole grains in your meals? The goal is to create awareness so that decisions can be made with knowledge, not perfection.

Setting reasonable and attainable goals for improvement is the next step after identifying patterns in your diet. These objectives ought to be incremental, focusing on tiny, steady improvements that, over time, can produce noteworthy outcomes. Week 1 is the time to start making positive adjustments to your diet that will lead to a heart-healthy lifestyle, such as cutting back on processed foods, eating more vegetables, or practicing mindful eating.

Creating Weekly Workout Schedules

Since exercise is essential for heart health, Week 1 is devoted to creating a realistic fitness schedule that fits your schedule. Recognizing that not everyone enjoys working out at the gym, the emphasis is on finding enjoyable activities that you can incorporate easily into your everyday routine.

Discover a variety of workouts, including at-home workouts and brisk walks, under the guidance of professional advice and instructions. The intention is to see physical activity as a source of enjoyment and general well-being rather than as a necessary chore. Workout regimens that can be tailored to meet a variety of fitness levels and tastes are offered, guaranteeing accessibility and enjoyment for those who want to lead an active lifestyle.

Exercise should be a habit. Consistency is crucial. The goal is to engage in things that you find personally fulfilling because this will increase the likelihood that you will maintain your habit over time.

Determining Heart-Healthy Objectives

Sustainable lifestyle changes require the establishment of specific, quantifiable, and achievable goals. The first week walks you through the process of selecting heart-healthy objectives that fit your particular requirements and ambitions. These objectives cover nutrition, physical activity, and overall health.

Think beyond just your physical well-being while creating goals. Emotional and mental health are essential to heart health. Goals may encompass stress reduction techniques, mindfulness practices, or fostering positive social connections. This all-encompassing method guarantees a thorough plan for heart health that touches every aspect of your life.

Objectives act as your own road map, providing guidance, inspiration, and a concrete way to track your development as you travel towards heart health.

By the time Week 1 ends, you will have a better grasp of your current routines in addition to a well-planned road map for the future. A well-rounded and sustainable approach to heart health is established by the exercise routines and heart-healthy goals, and by the self-assessment, which paves the way for positive dietary changes.

Week 1 is about building a strong foundation for the journey ahead, not about drastic changes. It's an odyssey of self-discovery, progress, and empowerment. Every intentional action made in Week 1 represents a step closer to living a healthier and more satisfying life.

Week 2: Investigating Heart-Healthy Substances

We go deeply into the world of heart-healthy ingredients in Week 2 of our path towards a heart-healthy lifestyle. This week is about comprehending, selecting, and using these components into your everyday life—it's not just about exploring. Here's a thorough analysis of all the important elements of Week 2:

Introduction to Nutrient-Rich Foods

Understanding what nutrient-rich foods are is crucial to starting a heart-healthy eating path. When compared to their calorie count, they are the nutritional powerhouses, providing a plethora of important vitamins, minerals, and other key nutrients. Week 2 serves as a guide to discovering and adding these nutritional powerhouses into your diet.

Start by acquainting yourself with a selection of nutrient-rich foods. The cornerstones of a heart-healthy diet are lean proteins, whole grains, colourful fruits and vegetables, and heart-healthy fats. Examine each area in detail to learn about its special advantages and how it affects general wellbeing.

For instance, green fruits and vegetables are high in antioxidants, which counteract oxidative stress and inflammation in the body—two critical factors associated to heart disease. Fibre from whole grains facilitates digestion and increases feelings of fullness. Fish and poultry, which are lean proteins, provide necessary amino acids without the saturated fats included in some red meats. Heart-healthy fats, such as those in almonds and avocados, help maintain a healthy cardiovascular system.

Week 2 makes sure you have the information to include these nutrient-dense foods in your meals in addition to making sure you are aware of them. This nutritional investigation is made concrete and accessible to your everyday life with helpful hints, recipe suggestions, and easy replacements.

Guide to Purchasing Heart-Healthy Pantry Essentials

Equipped with an understanding of nutrient-dense foods, Week 2 leads you to the next critical phase: purposefully navigating the grocery store. The Shopping Guide for

Heart-Healthy Pantry Staples is a complete tool to help you make heart-healthy decisions when you shop, not simply a list of items.

First and foremost, it's critical to comprehend the importance of reading food labels. In Week 2, we dissect food labels to assist you in understanding nutritional data, identifying hidden sources of bad fats and carbohydrates, and making heart-healthy selections.

The book presents you with a carefully chosen list of heart-healthy pantry essentials. Whole grains like brown rice and quinoa are the cornerstone of a heart-healthy kitchen. Legumes include fibre and plant-based protein, such as lentils and chickpeas. Nuts and seeds provide extra protein and good fats. The book also stresses the value of adding a range of herbs and spices to provide flavour without adding too much sodium.

Preparing Meals for Success

After obtaining heart-healthy products, the next thing to do is become an expert meal prepper. Week 2 acknowledges the rigours of contemporary living and offers a doable framework for meal planning ahead of time, so that heart-healthy options are easily included into your hectic routine.

Meal prep is about efficient and strategic planning, not about spending hours in the kitchen every day. The procedure is broken down into doable steps in Week 2. To begin, prepare ingredients ahead of time by chopping veggies, marinating meats, and dividing grains into serving sizes. This simplifies cooking and saves time during the workweek.

The weekly meal plans are made to be diverse, so you can expect a variety of tastes and textures to keep your meals interesting. A focus is on using a range of heart-healthy components to create a satisfying and delightful meal experience. We help you create balanced, nutrient-dense meals because we recognise how important variety is to maintaining a healthy diet.

Meal planning becomes an accessible and essential part of your routine thanks to the time-saving tricks and useful advice included with the meal prep programmes. By the end of the second week, you will have gained knowledge about heart-healthy ingredients and the ability to cook them into your weekly meals with ease. This will promote a heart-healthy lifestyle that is both pleasurable and long-lasting.

To sum up, Week 2 is about empowerment more than just exploration. It gives you the information and resources you need to choose, buy, and cook heart-healthy foods. This week lays the groundwork for a revolutionary and long-lasting path towards a heart-healthy lifestyle, from learning the nutritional value of foods to confidently navigating the grocery store and perfecting the art of meal prep.

Week 3: Try New Cooking Methods

Week 3 is a critical time in your journey to a heart-healthy lifestyle because we're going to be diving into the world of cooking. This week is devoted to attempting new culinary methods, adopting heart-healthy practices, experimenting with delectable substitutes for seasoning, and acquiring practical expertise through practice and cooking demonstrations. Now let's examine the specifics of Week 3:

Heart-Healthy Recipe Ideas

It's essential to comprehend how cooking techniques affect the nutritional value of your food in order to create a diet that promotes heart health. In Week 3, we break down the complexities of heart-healthy cooking techniques so that every dish you make benefits your general health.

Baking and Roasting: These techniques cook food using low heat, which reduces the requirement for additional fats. Baking and roasting help to maintain the natural flavors of food, including succulent vegetables and lean proteins, while also supporting heart health.

Steaming: Steaming is an easy yet efficient way to retain nutrients and maintain the natural colors and textures of your products. It's especially helpful for veggies, keeping them crunchy and full of vital nutrients.

Grilling: A great option for heart-healthy cooking, grilling imparts a smokey flavors without using an excessive amount of lipids. We provide you with instructions on how to create the ideal grill, maximizing flavor and reducing the production of dangerous substances.

Sautéing with Healthy Oils: Selecting heart-healthy oils, such as olive oil, improves the nutritional profile while also giving your food more depth through sautéing. To preserve their health benefits, we offer advice on how to choose the best oils and regulate cooking temperatures.

Poaching: This technique, which involves slowly cooking food in a simmering broth, is a great way to retain flavour and softness without using too much fat. It works especially well with fragile proteins like eggs and seafood.

In addition to improving the flavour of your food, knowing and using these cooking techniques can help you lead a heart-healthy lifestyle. Week Three provides you with the information to make well-informed decisions regarding your cooking methods through thorough explanations and useful advice.

Tasteful Substitutes for Seasoning

It's an art to enhance the flavor of your food without sacrificing heart health. We look at inventive methods to give your dishes more depth and flavor while reducing your reliance on salt and unhealthy condiments:

Herbs and Spices: Unleash the flavor-enhancing potential of natural ingredients. We explore the world of herbs and spices, each with their own special health advantages, from cumin and turmeric to basil and cilantro.

Citrus Zest and Juices: Citrus zest and juices give flavors a lift and add vitamin C and antioxidants. They also add a burst of freshness. Gain expertise in the art of adjusting the acidity level of your food.

Garlic and Onions: Rich in flavor and beneficial to the heart, these aromatic ingredients also impart robust flavors. Find out how to make the most of them and use the least amount of salt possible.

Vinegars: Adding a little vinegar to your food will give it a tangy kick. We discuss the different kinds of vinegars and how to use them in your cooking.

Homemade Sauces and Dressings: You can maintain ingredient control and steer clear of unhealthy fats and hidden sugars by making your own sauces and dressings. The third week offers easy-to-make but delicious recipes for making your own heart-healthy condiments.You'll discover that a world of flavour opens up as you experiment with these substitutes for seasoning, turning your heart-healthy journey into a culinary adventure as well as a health conscious one.

Cooking Practice and Demonstrations

Without practice, theory is insufficient. In addition to making sure you comprehend the fundamentals of heart-healthy cooking, Week 3 offers practice sessions and cooking demonstrations to give you practical experience.

Step-by-Step Examples: Learning visually is effective. Participate in cooking demonstrations that walk you through the process of preparing heart-healthy meals. These demos cover everything from roasting a chicken to sautéing veggies in the appropriate oils. They provide helpful advice.

Guided Practice Sessions: Use the guided practice sessions to put your newly acquired knowledge into practice. We give easy yet impactful dishes for you to attempt, using the cooking methods and seasoning choices taught during the week. These practical tasks are meant to increase your confidence and expertise in the kitchen.

By the end of Week 3, you won't only possess theoretical knowledge; you'll be a confident and skilled practitioner of heart-healthy cooking. The combination of informed choices in cooking methods and innovative seasoning alternatives empowers you to transform every meal into a delectable, healthy, and heart-conscious joy. Week 3 sets the scene for a lifetime of gastronomic enjoyment, illustrating that heart-healthy may also mean deliciously rewarding.

Week 4: Sustainable Practices for Long-Term Health

As we approach the completion of our 4-week journey toward a heart-healthy lifestyle, Week 4 is carefully planned to implant sustainable principles for long-term health. This week is not just about reaching a finish line but about building the groundwork for enduring well-being. In Week 4, we go into making a balanced meal plan, developing a realistic workout programme, and setting goals that pave the road for continued success. Let's break down the important components:

Creating a Balanced Meal Plan

Creating a balanced meal plan is at the basis of keeping a heart-healthy lifestyle. It's not about short-term remedies but about encouraging a style of eating that nourishes your body consistently. In Week 4, you will receive the tools and knowledge needed to construct a meal plan that meets your specific preferences, dietary limitations, and long-term goals.Start by revisiting the nutrient-rich meals covered in Week 2. These need to be the cornerstone of your diets, providing a wide range of vital elements and vitamins. Think about including a range of healthful grains, fruits, vegetables, lean meats, and heart-healthy fats in your regular diet. We offer helpful advice on mindful eating, controlling portion sizes, and adding tasty, heart-healthy ingredients to your meals.

Rather than rigid regulations, the focus is on fun and freedom. Meal plans should be flexible enough to fit your lifestyle, allowing for social gatherings and occasional indulgences. By the end of Week 4, you'll have a customized meal plan along with the know-how to adjust it to suit your changing needs.

Creating a Practical Workout Schedule

One thing that cannot be compromised for long-term heart health is physical activity. But maintaining a fitness regimen necessitates a practical and pleasurable strategy. The goal of week four is to assist you in creating a fitness regimen that fits into your daily schedule and will be consistent in the long run.

Think back on the drills and tasks performed throughout the first week. What struck a chord with you? What makes you happy and gives you a feeling of success? It might be a mix of recreational sports, at-home workouts, and brisk walks. Finding things that you truly enjoy will increase the likelihood that you'll remain with them.

Fitting your routine around your natural tendencies is important, regardless of whether you're an early riser or an evening worker. We also discuss the significance of adding cardiovascular workouts, flexibility exercises, and strength training to a well-rounded fitness regimen.

By the conclusion of Week 4, you will have an exercise regimen that works well for you on a daily basis. The idea is to see exercise as an essential component of your routine that enhances your general health rather than as a taxing chore.

Setting Objectives for Ongoing Achievement

After four weeks, the path to a heart-healthy lifestyle doesn't end; it's a continuous process that calls for continual drive and dedication. The fourth week's theme is goal-setting as a strategy for long-term success. Instead of putting arbitrary goals in place, we walk you through a deliberate process of choosing targets that match your changing dreams.

Think back on the objectives from Week 1. What strides have you made? What modifications are required? Make use of this introspection to establish new objectives that build upon your successes. To ensure that you feel a sense of accomplishment when you meet each milestone, your goals should be realistic, measurable, and explicit.

We present the idea of short- and long-term goals, stressing the value of acknowledging minor accomplishments along the road. Your objectives should include mental and emotional health in addition to nutrition and exercise. You use stress management techniques, mindfulness training, and building healthy relationships into your goal-setting process.

Week 4 offers advice on goal-setting as well as progress monitoring. Whether you use measurements, journals, or other techniques, regular evaluations keep you accountable and inspired. We also talk about how important it is to modify your goals as needed, understanding that flexibility is essential for reacting to the always shifting conditions of life.

Heart-Healthy Recipes

Breakfast Recipes

1. Vegan Date Muffins with Sweet Potatoes

Ingredients

A cup and a half of whole wheat flour

A teaspoon of baking powder

One teaspoon of ground cinnamon

Half a teaspoon of salt

1 1/2 cups of sweet potatoes, cooked

1/2 cup chopped pitted dates

Half a cup of almond milk without sugar

One-third cup pure maple syrup

Two tablespoons ground flaxseed

One teaspoon of vanilla extract

Guidelines:

Start the oven at 350°F, or 180°C.

Combine flour, baking powder, cinnamon, and salt in a sizable bowl.

Combine the sweet potato, dates, almond milk, flaxseed, maple syrup, and vanilla extract in a another bowl.

Stir just until mixed after adding the wet components to the dry ingredients.

Pour batter into a 12-cup muffin tray; bake for 20 to 25 minutes, or until toothpick inserted in center comes out clean.

After five minutes of cooling in the pan, move the food to a wire rack to finish cooling.

Nutritional value: High in potassium, which lowers blood pressure, as well as vitamins, minerals, and fiber.

2. Amaranth with Walnuts and Honey

Ingredients

One cup of amaranth

Two cups milk or water

One-half cup honey

Chopped walnuts, half a cup

One-fourth cup chia seeds

Guidelines:

Drain and rinse the amaranth with cool water.

Put the amaranth, milk or water, honey, and walnuts in a saucepan.

Bring to a boil, then lower heat and simmer until liquid is absorbed, about 20 minutes.

Turn off the heat and give it a few minutes to cool.

Add the chia seeds and stir until the mixture becomes thick.

Nutritional value: Rich in fibre, magnesium, and copper, amaranth promotes heart health.

3. Almonds, Berries, and Bananas Smoothie

Ingredients

One-half cup almond milk

Half a cup of Greek yoghurt

1/2 cup of mixed berries, including blackberries, raspberries, strawberries, and blueberries

One half banana

One tablespoon honey

1 tablespoon of ground cinnamon

Guidelines:

Blend together almond milk, Greek yoghurt, banana, mixed berries, honey, and cinnamon in a blender.

Blend till creamy and smooth.

Nutritional value: Probiotics and protein from Greek yoghurt help maintain digestive health.

4. Soft-cooked egg served with orange slices on whole wheat toast

Ingredients

One piece of whole wheat bread

One egg, soft-boiled

Half a cup of orange slices

One tablespoon of avocado

To taste, add salt and pepper.

Guidelines:

Make whole wheat toast.

Bring a saucepan of water to a boil, then cook the egg for four to five minutes, or until the yolk sets but the whites are still runny.

Peel and drain the egg.

Place avocado, orange slices, and soft-boiled egg on top of the toast.

Season to taste with salt and pepper.

Nutritional value: Eggs and whole wheat bread are excellent providers of heart-healthy lipids and fiber

5. Whole-grain pita pocket with banana and peanut butter

Ingredients

One pita pocket with whole grains

2 tablespoons peanut butter, or substitute (almond butter, for example)

Half a banana, cut

Guidelines:

Spread the nut butter inside the pita pocket after opening it.

Close the pita pocket after adding the banana slices.

Nutritional value: Rich in fiber and heart-healthy fats, peanut butter is a good source of both

6. Tofu Scramble with Spices

Ingredients

One block of crumbled and pressed extra-firm tofu

Half a cup of finely chopped onion

Half a cup of bell pepper, chopped

Half a cup of chopped tomatoes

One tablespoon of olive oil

1-tablespoon curry powder

To taste, add salt and pepper.

Guidelines:

Combine the crumbled tofu, onion, bell pepper, and tomato in a big bowl.

In a big skillet over medium heat, warm the olive oil.

Add the tofu mixture and cook, stirring occasionally, until the vegetables become soft, about 4–5 minutes.

Add the pepper, salt, and curry powder and stir.

Nutritional value: Tofu is a good source of protein and healthy fats, which support heart health

7. California Walnut and Apple Bircher Pots

Ingredients

1/2 cup rolled oats

1 cup apple juice or milk

1/4 cup chopped walnuts

1/4 cup raisins

1/4 cup unsweetened shredded coconut

1/4 cup Greek yogurt

One tablespoon honey

Guidelines:

In a bowl, mix together oats, apple juice or milk, walnuts, raisins, and shredded coconut.

Cover and refrigerate for at least 4 hours or overnight.

In the morning, stir in Greek yogurt and honey.

Nutritional value: Oats and walnuts are good sources of fiber and healthy

8. Overnight oats

Ingredients

1/2 cup rolled oats

Half a cup of almond milk without sugar

Half a mashed banana

One tablespoon of chia seeds

One tablespoon honey

Guidelines:

Combine oats, almond milk, mashed banana, chia seeds, and honey in a jar or other container.

Place a lid on and chill for the night.

In the morning, stir and add toppings of your choice, such as fresh fruit or nuts.

Nutritional value: Oats and chia seeds are good sources of fiber and healthy fats, which support heart health

9. Healthy Pancakes

Ingredients

1 cup whole wheat flour

1 tbsp baking powder

1/4 tsp salt

1 cup unsweetened almond milk

1 egg

One tablespoon honey

One teaspoon of vanilla extract

Guidelines:

In a large bowl, whisk together flour, baking powder, and salt.

In a separate bowl, stir together almond milk, egg, honey, and vanilla extract.

Stir just until mixed after adding the wet components to the dry ingredients.

Heat a non-stick skillet over medium heat.

Pour 1/4 cup of batter onto the skillet and cook until bubbles form on the surface, then turn and cook until golden brown.

Repeat with remaining batter.

Nutritional value: Whole wheat flour and almond milk are wonderful sources of fiber and healthy fats, which improve heart health

10. Mushroom hash with poached eggs

Ingredients

One tablespoon of olive oil

1/2 onion, chopped

2 cups sliced mushrooms

1/2 red bell pepper, chopped

Half a chopped green bell pepper

1/2 tsp of paprika smoked

To taste, add salt and pepper.

Two stolen eggs

Guidelines:

In a big skillet over medium heat, warm the olive oil.

Add onion and cook until softened, 2 to 3 minutes.

Add the smoked paprika, red and green bell peppers, mushrooms, salt, and pepper.

Cook, stirring regularly, until veggies are soft, 5 to 7 minutes.

Top with poached eggs and serve.

Nutritional value: Rich in fibre and antioxidants, mushrooms promote heart health

1. Minestrone Soup

Ingredients

One tablespoon of olive oil

1 onion, chopped

2 garlic cloves, minced

2 carrots, chopped

2 celery stalks, chopped

Diced tomatoes, one can

4 cups vegetable broth

1 can kidney beans, drained and rinsed

1 cup chopped kale

1 tsp dried basil

To taste, add salt and pepper.

Guidelines:

Heat olive oil in a big pot over medium heat.

Add onion and garlic and simmer for 2-3 minutes, until softened.

Add the celery and carrots and simmer for 5 to 7 minutes, or until soft.

Add the kidney beans, kale, basil, diced tomatoes, vegetable broth, salt, and pepper.

Bring to a boil, then simmer for 20 to 30 minutes on low heat.

Nutritional value: Rich in fibre, vitamins, and minerals, minestrone soup promotes heart health

2. Vegetable Salad

Ingredients

Mixed greens, such as spinach, kale and rocket

A variety of vegetables, such as beets, broccoli, Brussel sprouts, and sweet potatoes

Nuts or legumes, such as walnuts, almonds, and chickpeas

Dressing made with extra virgin olive oil and vinegar

Guidelines:

Begin with a mixed greens bed.

Add your preferred nuts or legumes along with the veggies.

Drizzle with a dressing made of extra virgin olive oil and vinegar.

Nutritional value: Fibre, vitamins, and minerals, which promote heart health, can be found in a salad made with mixed greens and a variety of vegetables

3. Turkey Wrap

Ingredients

One whole-grain tortilla

Two ounces of sliced turkey breast

1/4 sliced avocado

1/4 cup of carrots, shredded

1/4 cup baby spinach

One tablespoon of hummus

Guidelines:

Lay the wrap flat and sprinkle hummus on it.

Include the avocado, baby spinach, shredded carrots, and turkey breast.

After rolling the wrap, cut it in half.

Nutritional value: Fibre, protein, and heart-healthy fats are all present in a turkey wrap made with whole-grain wrap and veggies

4. Tuna Sandwich

Ingredients

Two slices of bread with grains.

2 ounces of drained canned tuna

1-tablespoon Greek yoghurt

Chopped celery, one tablespoon

One tablespoon finely minced red onion

One tablespoon finely chopped parsley

To taste, add salt and pepper.

Guidelines:

Make wholegrain toast.

Combine the tuna, Greek yoghurt, parsley, celery, red onion, and salt and pepper in a bowl.

Spread one slice of bread with the tuna mixture, then cover it with the second slice.

Nutritional value: Greek yoghurt, whole-grain bread, and tuna make a heart-healthy sandwich that's high in protein and heart-healthy fats

5. Grain Bowl

Ingredients

Cooked whole grains, such as farro, brown rice, and quinoa

A variety of vegetables, such as tomatoes, bell peppers, black beans, cucumbers, and red onions

A variety of herbs, such as basil, parsley, and cilantro

Dressing made with extra virgin olive oil and vinegar

Guidelines:

Begin by spreading cooked whole grains on a bed.

Incorporate your preferred herbs and veggies.

Drizzle with a dressing made of extra virgin olive oil and vinegar.

Nutritional value: Heart health is supported by the fibre, vitamins, and minerals found in a grain bowl with whole grains and a variety of vegetables

6. Beetroot Hummus

Ingredients

1 can chickpeas, drained and rinsed

1/2 cup finely chopped cooked beetroot

One minced clove of garlic

2 tbsp tahini

Two tablespoons of lemon juice

1 tbsp extra-virgin olive oil

To taste, add salt and pepper.

Guidelines:

Put the chickpeas, tahini, lemon juice, garlic, beetroot, and olive oil in a food processor.

Process until smooth and creamy.

Season to taste with salt and pepper.

Nutritional value: Rich in fibre and antioxidants, beetroot promotes heart health.

7. Garlic Beef Stir-Fried with Peppers

Ingredients

1 tablespoon of olive oil

Slicing 1 pound of beef sirloin

One sliced red bell pepper

One sliced green bell pepper

1 tbsp grated ginger

Two minced garlic cloves

Two tablespoons of soy sauce

One tablespoon honey

To taste, add salt and pepper.

Guidelines:

In a large skillet, heat the vegetable oil over high heat.

Cook the beef sirloin for two to three minutes, or until browned.

Add the ginger, garlic, and bell peppers, both red and green, and simmer for 2 to 3 minutes, or until the vegetables are soft.

Add the honey, soy sauce, salt, and pepper and stir.

Nutritional value: Iron and protein from beef sirloin are excellent for heart health.

8. Pea Pancakes Miniature

Ingredients

One cup of thawed frozen peas

One-half cup of whole wheat flour

Half a cup of almond milk without sugar

One egg

One tablespoon of olive oil

To taste, add salt and pepper.

Guidelines:

Place the peas, almond milk, whole wheat flour, egg, olive oil, salt, and pepper in a blender.

Blend till creamy and smooth.

A nonstick skillet should be heated to medium heat.

Transfer 1 tablespoon of batter to the skillet, let it bubble on top, then turn it over and continue cooking it until it turns golden brown.

Continue with the leftover batter.

Nutritional value: Whole wheat flour, peas, and vitamins are excellent providers of fibre, vitamins, and minerals that promote heart health.

9. Smoky Chipotle Adzuki Bean Chilli

Ingredients

One tablespoon of olive oil

One chopped onion

Two minced garlic cloves

One chopped red bell pepper

One sliced green bell pepper

One can of rinsed and drained Adzuki beans

One can of chopped tomatocs

One tablespoon of chipotle in adobo sauce

1 tsp of paprika with smoke

To taste, add salt and pepper.

Guidelines:

In a large pot set over medium heat, warm the olive oil.

Cook the onion and garlic for two to three minutes, or until they are tender.

Cook the red and green bell peppers for five to seven minutes, or until they are soft.

Stir in diced tomatoes, smoked paprika, chipotle in adobo sauce, adzuki beans, and salt and pepper.

Bring to a boil, then simmer for 20 to 30 minutes on low heat.

Nutritional value: Rich in fibre and protein, adzuki beans promote heart health.

10. Quinoa Bowl with Salmon

Ingredients

A cup of prepared quinoa

4 ounces of cooked salmon

Half of an avocado, cut

1/4 cup of cucumber, chopped

1/4 cup of red onion, chopped

One tablespoon of extra virgin olive oil

1-tablespoon lemon juice

To taste, add salt and pepper.

Guidelines:

Put the cooked quinoa, salmon, avocado, cucumber, and red onion in a bowl.

Drizzle with lemon juice and extra virgin olive oil.

Season to taste with salt and pepper.

Nutritional value: Quinoa is a rich source of fibre and protein, and salmon is a good source of omega-3 fatty acids, which support heart health.

Dinner Recipes

1. Sardines and Cherry Tomatoes over Spaghetti

Ingredients

Eight ounces of whole-grain spaghetti

One tablespoon of olive oil

Two minced garlic cloves

One can of flaked and drained sardines

Half a pint of cherry tomatoes

1/4 cup of parsley, chopped

To taste, add salt and pepper.

Guidelines:

Prepare pasta as directed on the package.

In a big skillet over medium heat, warm the olive oil.

Cook the garlic for one to two minutes, or until fragrant.

Cook the cherry tomatoes and sardines for two to three minutes, or until well heated.

Add the cooked spaghetti, salt, pepper, and parsley and stir.

Nutritional value: Sardines and whole-grain spaghetti are excellent providers of heart-healthy lipids and fibre, both of which promote heart health

2. Hummus Made with Beetroot

Ingredients

One can of washed and drained chickpeas

1/2 cup finely chopped cooked beetroot

One minced clove of garlic

Two tablespoons of tahini

Two tablespoons of lemon juice

One tablespoon of extra virgin olive oil

To taste, add salt and pepper.

Guidelines:

Put the chickpeas, tahini, lemon juice, garlic, beetroot, and olive oil in a food processor.

Process till creamy and smooth.

Season to taste with salt and pepper.

Nutritional value: Rich in fibre and antioxidants, beetroot promotes heart health..

3. Garlic Beef Stir-Fried with Peppers

Ingredients

1 tablespoon of olive oil

Slicing 1 pound of beef sirloin

One sliced red bell pepper

One sliced green bell pepper

One tablespoon grated ginger

Two minced garlic cloves

Two tablespoons of soy sauce

One tablespoon honey

To taste, add salt and pepper.

Guidelines:

In a large skillet, heat the vegetable oil over high heat.

Cook the beef sirloin for two to three minutes, or until browned.

Add the ginger, garlic, and bell peppers, both red and green, and simmer for 2 to 3 minutes, or until the vegetables are soft.

Add the honey, soy sauce, salt, and pepper and stir.

Nutritional value: Iron and protein from beef sirloin are excellent for heart health..

4. Spicy Stew of Lentils

Ingredient

One tablespoon of olive oil

One chopped onion

Two minced garlic cloves

2 sliced carrots

Two sliced celery stalks

Diced tomatoes, one can

Four cups broth made of vegetables

1 cup of lentils, dried

1 tsp of paprika with smoke

To taste, add salt and pepper.

Guidelines:

In a large pot set over medium heat, warm the olive oil.

Cook the onion and garlic for two to three minutes, or until they are tender.

Add the celery and carrots and simmer for 5 to 7 minutes, or until soft.

Add the lentils, smoked paprika, diced tomatoes, vegetable broth, salt, and pepper.

Bring to a boil, then simmer for 20 to 30 minutes on low heat.

Nutritional value: Rich in fibre and protein, lentils promote heart health.

5. Tuna Salsa with Baked Sweet Potatoes

Ingredients

Four candied sweet potatoes

Two drained tuna cans

1/2 chopped red onion

1/2 chopped red bell pepper

Half a chopped green bell pepper

1/4 cup of parsley, chopped

Two tablespoons of extra virgin olive oil

Two tablespoons of lemon juice

To taste, add salt and pepper.

Guidelines:

Set oven temperature to 200°C/400°F.

Arrange the sweet potatoes on a baking sheet after piercing them with a fork.

Bake until soft, 45 to 50 minutes.

Combine the tuna, parsley, olive oil, lemon juice, red onion, and green and red bell peppers in a bowl. Season with salt and pepper.

Cover roasted sweet potatoes with tuna salsa.

Nutritional value: Heart health is supported by the high fibre and heart-healthy fat content of sweet potatoes and tuna..

6. Fish Stew

Ingredients

One tablespoon of olive oil

One chopped onion

Two minced garlic cloves

One chopped red bell pepper

One sliced green bell pepper

Diced tomatoes, one can

Four cups of fish stock

One-pound white fish fillets, sliced into pieces

1/4 cup of parsley, chopped

To taste, add salt and pepper.

Guidelines:

In a large pot set over medium heat, warm the olive oil.

Cook the onion and garlic for two to three minutes, or until they are tender.

Cook the red and green bell peppers for five to seven minutes, or until they are soft.

Include the diced tomatoes and fish stock; heat until boiling.

For ten to fifteen minutes, simmer over low heat.

Cook the white fish fillets for 5 to 7 minutes, or until the fish is well done.

Add the pepper, salt, and parsley and stir.

Nutritional value: Omega-3 fatty acids and protein are abundant in white fish fillets, supporting heart health.

7. Curried lentils

Ingredients

1 tablespoon of olive oil

One chopped onion

Two minced garlic cloves

2 sliced carrots

Two sliced celery stalks

Diced tomatoes, one can

Four cups broth made of vegetables

1 cup of lentils, dried

1-tablespoon curry powder

To taste, add salt and pepper.

Guidelines:

In a big pot, warm up the vegetable oil over medium heat.

Cook the onion and garlic for two to three minutes, or until they are tender.

Add the celery and carrots and simmer for 5 to 7 minutes, or until soft.

Add lentils, chopped tomatoes, curry powder, salt, and pepper along with the vegetable broth.

Bring to a boil, then simmer for 20 to 30 minutes on low heat.

Nutritional value: Rich in fibre and protein, lentils promote heart health.

8. Kebabs with Chicken

Ingredients

One-pound chicken breast, sliced into pieces

One chopped onion

One sliced green bell pepper

One chopped red bell pepper

One chopped courgette

1/4 cup of halved cherry tomatoes

1/4 cup finely sliced red onion

One-fourth cup balsamic vinegar

One-fourth cup olive oil

Two minced garlic cloves

One teaspoon dried oregano

To taste, add salt and pepper.

Guidelines:

Combine the chicken, onion, zucchini, cherry tomatoes, red onion, green and red peppers, balsamic vinegar, olive oil, garlic and oregano in a sizable bowl.

Marinate in the refrigerator for at least 30 minutes.

Set grill's temperature to medium-high.

Grill the kebabs until they are cooked through, about 2 to 3 minutes per side.

Nutritional value: Lean chicken breast is high in protein and low in fat, both of which are beneficial to heart health.

9. Mediterranean Quinoa Salad

Ingredients

A cup of prepared quinoa

Half a cup of cooked lentils

1/2 cup of tomatoes, diced

1/2 cup diced cucumber

1/2 cup of red onion, chopped

1/4 cup Kalamata olives, pitted and halved

1/4 cup crumbled feta cheese

1/4 cup finely chopped fresh parsley

1/4 cup finely chopped fresh mint

1/4 cup finely chopped fresh basil

One-fourth cup lemon juice

One tablespoon red wine vinegar

One tablespoon of extra virgin olive oil

To taste, add salt and pepper.

Guidelines:

Combine the cooked quinoa, cooked chickpeas, olive oil, lemon juice, red wine vinegar, tomatoes, cucumbers, red onions, feta cheese, parsley, mint, and basil in a big bowl.

Season to taste with salt and pepper.

Nutritional value: Rich in fiber and protein, quinoa and chickpeas promote heart health.

10. Stir-fried tofu

Ingredients

1 tablespoon of olive oil

One block of pressed and cubed extra-firm tofu

One chopped onion

One minced clove of garlic

One sliced bell pepper

Slicing one cup of mushrooms

1/4 cup soy sauce with low sodium

One tablespoon cornflour

To taste, add salt and pepper.

Guidelines:

In a large skillet set over medium heat, heat the vegetable oil.

Cook the tofu for two to three minutes, or until it browns.

Cook the bell pepper, mushrooms, onion, and garlic for 5 to 7 minutes, or until the vegetables are soft.

Combine the corn flour and soy sauce in a small bowl.

Drizzle the tofu and veggies with the sauce, tossing to coat.

Simmer for a further one to two minutes, or until the sauce gets thicker.

Nutritional value: Rich in heart-healthy fats and protein, tofu is a good source of both.

Smoothie Recipes

1. Completely Blended Berry Smoothie

Ingredients

One cup of mixed berries (cranberries, raspberries, blueberries, and strawberries)

1/2 cup soy, dairy, or almond milk

One banana

One cup of finely chopped spinach

One tablespoon of flax seed

One teaspoon grated ginger

One teaspoon of mint leaves

One teaspoon of lemon juice

Taste of honey

Guidelines:

Blend the berries, milk, banana, spinach, flax seed, ginger, mint leaves, and lemon juice together in a blender.

Taste and add honey.

Blend until no lumps remain.

Nutritional value: Rich in fibre and antioxidants that are vital for heart health, berries are a superfood. In addition, this smoothie has a lot of vitamins, minerals, and excellent fats

2. Fruit Smoothie

Ingredients

One cup of de-stemmed strawberries

Half a cup blueberries

One peeled orange

One cup sliced, peeled, and seeded papaya

1 cup soy milk

Half a cup of ice cubes

Guidelines:

Place all of the fruits, ice, and soy milk in a blender.

Blend until no lumps remain.

Nutritious value: The fruits in this smoothie are a great source of vitamins, minerals, and antioxidants, and the soy milk adds heart-healthy fats and proteins.

3. Breakfast Smoothie

Ingredients

Half a cup of frozen pineapple

Half a cup of frozen mango

One half banana

Half a cup of spinach

Half a cup of Greek yoghurt

One-half cup almond milk

One tablespoon of chia seeds

Guidelines:

Blend together the banana, spinach, Greek yoghurt, almond milk, chia seeds, pineapple, and mango in a blender.

Blend until no lumps remain.

Nutritional value: Probiotics, fibre, and protein in this smoothie are excellent for heart health.

4. Grid-Banana Smoothie

Ingredients

One sliced ripe banana

One-third cup of vanilla yoghurt

Half a cup of chilled apple juice

Half a teaspoon of honey

1/2 tsp finely chopped ginger

Guidelines:

Blend together the banana, apple juice, ginger, honey, vanilla yoghurt, and apple juice in a blender.

Blend until no lumps remain.

Nutritional value: Probiotics, antioxidants, and potassium are all found in good amounts in this smoothie, all of which promote heart health.

5. Iced Banana Turmeric Smoothie

Ingredients

One huge frozen banana

One cup of almond milk without sugar

Half a teaspoon ground turmeric

Half a teaspoon ground cinnamon

Guidelines:

Blend together the frozen banana, almond milk, cinnamon, and turmeric in a blender.

Blend until no lumps remain.

Nutritional value: The anti-inflammatory qualities of turmeric, fibre, and potassium in this smoothie promote heart health.

6. Sweetheart Hazelnut Chocolate

Ingredients

One cup of almond milk without sugar

Half a cup of Greek yoghurt

1 tablespoon powdered unsweetened cocoa

1/4 cup of almonds

One half banana

One tablespoon honey

Guidelines:

Blend together the Greek yoghurt, almond milk, hazelnuts, banana, honey, and cocoa powder in a blender.

Blend until no lumps remain.

Nutritional value: Rich in heart-healthy fats, protein, and antioxidants, this smoothie is a great source of these nutrients.

7. Blueberry, Banana, and Strawberry Smoothie

Ingredients

Half a cup of strawberries

Half a cup blueberries

One banana

Half a cup of spinach

One-half cup almond milk

Half a cup of Greek yoghurt

One tablespoon honey

Guidelines:

Blend together the almond milk, Greek yoghurt, honey, banana, spinach, blueberries, and strawberries in a blender.

Blend until no lumps remain.

Nutritional value: Probiotics, vitamins, minerals, and antioxidants are abundant in this smoothie and improve heart health.

8. Green Pineapple Smoothie

Ingredients

One cup of pineapple, frozen

Half a cup of spinach

One-half cup kale

Half a cup of coconut water

Fresh ginger, 1/2 inch

Half an inch of newly harvested turmeric

Juiced half a lemon

Guidelines:

Place the frozen pineapple, kale, spinach, ginger, turmeric, and lemon juice in a blender.

Blend until no lumps remain.

Nutritional value: The anti-inflammatory qualities of turmeric and ginger, as well as the vitamins and minerals in this smoothie, improve heart health.

9. Spinach and Mixed Berry Smoothie

Ingredients

1/2 cup of mixed berries, including raspberries, blueberries, and strawberries

One half banana

One cup of spinach

One-half cup almond milk

Half a cup of Greek yoghurt

One tablespoon of chia seeds

Guidelines:

Blend together the mixed berries, banana, spinach, Greek yoghurt, almond milk, and chia seeds in a blender.

Blend until no lumps remain.

Nutritional value: Probiotics, fibre, and antioxidants found in this smoothie help to maintain heart health.

10. Watermelon Smoothie

Ingredients

Two cups cubed watermelon

Half a cup of strawberries

Half a cup of Greek yoghurt

Half a cup of coconut water

Half a cup of ice

One tablespoon honey

Guidelines:

Place the watermelon, strawberries, Greek yoghurt, ice, honey, and coconut water in a blender.

Blend until no lumps remain.

Nutritional value: This smoothie is a wonderful source of water, vitamins, minerals, and probiotics, which improve heart health.

Conclusion

As we reach the final chapter of "The Low Cholesterol Cookbook and Action Plan," we want to convey our heartfelt gratitude to each and every one of you. We appreciate you letting us accompany you on your path to a heart-healthy lifestyle. Sharing these pages with you and guiding you through the investigation of wholesome meals, useful advice, and sustainable practices has been an honour and a privilege.

It's admirable how dedicated you are to living a heart-healthy life. We hope that the information you learn from these pages will help you on your continuous path to wellbeing. May your heart pulse with energy and may all of your decisions lead to health and happiness as you move into the future.

If you've found value in this book, we respectfully ask for your cooperation in sharing your experience. Your opinions and suggestions may serve as inspiration for those who are pursuing a similar course. Think about posting a review on Amazon. Your words have the ability to help other readers make wise choices and start their own heart-healthy journeys.

Has there been a specific recipe that you use often? Did the meal planning advice completely alter your routine? Your knowledge can help others follow their own path and build a community of people who are heart health advocates. You become an inspiration to others who may be just beginning their journey by sharing your experiences.

We want you to consider how this book has affected your life and to tell the world about it. Your endorsements and reviews are more than just words on a screen; they are sparks that have the power to inspire good deeds in other people's lives.

I want to thank you one more for joining me on this amazing adventure. I hope your heart keeps beating in a healthy rhythm and that taking care of your health gives you the energy to live a vibrant life.